MIND DIET GUIDE BOOK

Foods that Boost and Preserve Brain Health: The MIND Diet

REX LEWIS

Table of Contents

Introduction

The MIND diet, short for "Mediterranean-DASH Diet Intervention for Neurodegenerative Delay," is a nutritional strategy aimed at enhancing brain health and lowering the likelihood of neurodegenerative disorders, specifically Alzheimer's disease. The MIND diet, created by academics Martha Clare Morris and her colleagues at Rush University Medical Center in Chicago, is a combination of the Mediterranean and DASH diets. Both of these diets have been linked to numerous health advantages.

The main emphasis of the MIND diet is on nutrients that are thought to enhance cognitive performance and safeguard the brain against age-related deterioration. The diet prioritizes the intake of foods that are rich in nutrients that have been associated with beneficial impacts on brain function. These encompass a diverse range of fruits, vegetables, whole grains, nuts, seeds, lean proteins, and specific types of fats. In addition, the MIND diet advises restricting the consumption of foods that could potentially harm cognitive health, such as processed meals, red meat, butter, and sweets.

The MIND diet consists of several essential elements:

• Consuming leafy green vegetables such as kale, spinach, and broccoli on a regular basis provides a high amount of vitamins and antioxidants.

• Berries, particularly blueberries and strawberries, are highlighted for their abundant anthocyanins, which are substances linked to cognitive advantages.

• **Nuts:** Addition of almonds and walnuts, which contribute beneficial fats, vitamins, and minerals.

• Opt for whole grains such as quinoa, brown rice, and oats, as they include both fiber and essential nutrients.

Regularly consuming fish, especially fatty fish such as salmon, provides omega-3 fatty acids that are advantageous for brain function.

• Incorporating beans and legumes into the diet for their high fiber and protein levels.

• **Poultry:** Consume a moderate amount of poultry, such as chicken or turkey, as a source of low-fat protein.

• Olive oil is used as the main source of fat because it is linked to the health of the heart and brain.

• **Wine:** It is recommended to consume red wine in moderation due to its content of resveratrol, a chemical that has been associated with cognitive advantages.

• Decreasing the consumption of processed meals, sugary treats, butter, and red meat.

The MIND diet is not a rigid routine, but rather offers broad principles for selecting healthier food options. Although continuous research is being conducted on the MIND diet, several studies indicate that adhering to this dietary pattern may be linked to a reduced likelihood of acquiring Alzheimer's disease and age-related cognitive decline. It is crucial to acknowledge that people may have different reactions to dietary interventions, and it is recommended to seek guidance from a healthcare practitioner or a qualified dietitian before making substantial modifications to one's diet.

CHAPTER ONE
What is the MIND Diet?

The MIND diet, acronym for "Mediterranean-DASH Diet Intervention for Neurodegenerative Delay," is a specific eating plan designed to enhance brain health and lower the likelihood of neurodegenerative disorders, specifically Alzheimer's disease. This diet is a combination of two widely recognized and extensively researched eating plans: the Mediterranean diet and the DASH (Dietary Approaches to Stop Hypertension) diet. The MIND diet was formulated by Martha Clare Morris and her colleagues at Rush University Medical Center in Chicago.

The MIND diet encompasses several important characteristics and principles:

• The MIND diet places importance on consuming foods that have been linked to improvements in cognitive function. The items that fall within this category are fruits, vegetables, nuts, berries, whole grains, fish, chicken, and olive oil.

• Berries, particularly blueberries and strawberries, are emphasized in the MIND diet because they contain a high amount of antioxidants and chemicals that may enhance brain function.

• Consuming leafy greens, such as kale, spinach, and broccoli, on a regular basis provides a high amount of vitamins and minerals.

• **Nuts and Seeds:** Incorporating nuts, namely walnuts, and seeds into the diet is beneficial due to their provision of nourishing fats and nutrients associated with cognitive well-being.

• Opt for whole grains instead than refined grains, as they include fiber and vital minerals.

Consuming fish, especially fatty fish such as salmon, is beneficial for cognitive health due to its high content of omega-3 fatty acids.

• Incorporate a moderate amount of poultry and, if preferred, red wine into the diet.

- Decrease the consumption of red meat, butter, sweets, and processed foods, as these items have been linked to potential adverse impacts on cognitive health.

The MIND diet is moderately permissive and permits freedom in food selection. It is intended to be a practical and enduring strategy for nourishing the brain over an extended period of time. Although research on the MIND diet is still developing, certain studies indicate that following this dietary pattern may be linked to a decreased likelihood of cognitive decline and Alzheimer's disease. Prior to making substantial alterations to your diet, particularly if you have specific health problems or diseases, it is crucial to get guidance from a healthcare expert or a qualified dietitian.

Importance of Brain-Healthy Diets

Diets that promote brain health are essential for enhancing cognitive performance, preserving mental clarity, and minimizing the likelihood of neurodegenerative disorders. There are numerous significant reasons that emphasize the need of choosing a diet that promotes brain health:

• Nutrient Support: The brain necessitates a diverse range of nutrients to operate at its highest level of efficiency. Foods that are abundant in nutrients, such as fruits, vegetables, whole grains, nuts, seeds, and fatty fish, include vital vitamins, minerals, antioxidants, and omega-3 fatty acids that promote brain function.

- Cognitive Function: Consuming a nutritionally balanced diet helps improve cognitive function, which includes abilities such as memory retention, concentration, and problem-solving proficiency. Specific nutrients, such as antioxidants and omega-3 fatty acids, have been associated with enhanced cognitive function and a decreased likelihood of cognitive deterioration.

• Certain foods exhibit neuroprotective characteristics, which means they can safeguard the brain from damage caused by oxidative stress, inflammation, and other factors linked to aging and neurodegenerative illnesses. Some examples of nutritious foods are berries, leafy greens, almonds, and fatty fish.

• Studies indicate that adhering to a diet that promotes brain health can decrease the likelihood of developing neurodegenerative disorders like Alzheimer's disease, Parkinson's disease, and dementia. Specific eating habits, such as following the Mediterranean diet and the MIND diet, have been linked to a lower occurrence of various illnesses.

• The cardiovascular system's well-being is intricately connected to the well-being of the brain. A heart-healthy diet, which includes a variety of fruits, vegetables, whole grains, and healthy fats, can also have positive effects on the brain. This type of food promotes good blood circulation and lowers the chances of illnesses like stroke, which can harm the brain.

• Diet has the ability to impact mood and mental well-being via regulating emotions. Consuming foods that are rich in nutrients and keeping blood sugar levels steady might aid in mood regulation and decrease the likelihood of developing illnesses such as sadness and anxiety.

• The brain necessitates a consistent provision of energy in order to operate with optimal efficiency. Whole grains provide complex carbs, which, when combined with healthy fats and protein, supply the brain with long-lasting energy, promoting focus and mental alertness.

• In terms of both cognitive health and overall well-being, adopting a brain-healthy diet has positive effects on one's overall health and lifespan. Several foods that promote brain health also enhance the immune system, maintain a balanced metabolism, and lower the likelihood of chronic conditions like diabetes and obesity.

To summarize, placing importance on consuming a diet that is abundant in foods that are high in nutrients, antioxidants, omega-3 fatty acids, and other nutrients that enhance brain function can have significant impacts on cognitive abilities, brain health, and general state of being. Engaging in well-informed dietary decisions and embracing a lifestyle that promotes brain health can effectively bolster long-term cognitive well-being and overall quality of life.

CHAPTER TWO
The Science behind the MIND Diet

The MIND diet is founded on scientific research that has examined the correlation between nutrition and cognitive well-being. Although the field of nutritional neuroscience is constantly changing, multiple studies provide evidence for the potential advantages of the MIND diet in enhancing brain health. The MIND diet is supported by several fundamental principles in scientific research:

• The MIND diet prioritizes the consumption of foods that are abundant in antioxidants, such as berries and leafy greens, in order to provide neuroprotection. Antioxidants aid in the fight against oxidative stress, a biological process associated with the aging process and the development of neurological disorders. Berries, specifically, have been linked to cognitive advantages because of their elevated concentrations of flavonoids and other substances with antioxidant characteristics.

• **Omega-3 Fatty Acids:** Fatty fish, which is commonly included in the MIND diet, provides omega-3 fatty acids. These indispensable fatty acids are vital for maintaining brain health, as they play a critical role in the formation of cell membranes and possess anti-inflammatory characteristics. Omega-3 fatty acids, including docosahexaenoic acid (DHA), have been identified as having a significant impact on cognitive function and perhaps serving as a safeguard against cognitive decline.

• Whole grains, which are an important part of the MIND diet, contain complex carbohydrates and vital nutrients that promote overall well-being and cognitive function. Studies indicate that consuming a diet abundant in whole grains may be linked to improved cognitive function and a decreased likelihood of experiencing cognitive decline.

• The MIND diet emphasizes the consumption of nutrient-dense foods that include high levels of vitamins and minerals necessary for optimal brain function. Examples of nutrient-dense choices include of verdant vegetables, nuts, and seeds. These food items enhance overall nutritional well-being and might exert beneficial impacts on cognitive health.

• The MIND diet advises restricting the consumption of inflammatory foods, such as red meat and processed foods. Neurodegenerative illnesses are among the health issues that are linked to chronic inflammation. The MIND diet tries to foster brain health by advocating for an anti-inflammatory diet.

- The MIND diet recommends consuming red wine in moderation due to its resveratrol content, which has the ability to preserve the brain. Nevertheless, it is crucial to acknowledge that excessive alcohol intake can have detrimental impacts on one's health, and the key to avoiding such consequences lies in practicing moderation.

- **Research Findings:** Studies have investigated the correlation between adherence to the MIND diet and cognitive outcomes. A study conducted at Rush University Medical Center, where the MIND diet was designed, has demonstrated that individuals who closely adhered to the diet reported a decelerated pace of cognitive decline and a decreased risk of developing Alzheimer's disease, in comparison to those who did not adhere to the diet as rigorously.

Although the scientific evidence supporting the MIND diet is encouraging, it is important to acknowledge that research in this area is still ongoing, and individual reactions to dietary patterns can differ. In addition, adhering to a well-rounded healthy lifestyle, which involves consistent physical exercise and mental engagement, enhances the advantages of a diet that promotes brain health. Prior to implementing substantial modifications to your dietary habits, it is recommended to seek advice from healthcare specialists or registered dietitians in order to receive specialized recommendations tailored to your health condition and specific requirements.

Understanding Neurodegenerative Diseases

Neurodegenerative illnesses refer to a collection of disorders marked by the gradual deterioration of the structure and operation of the nervous system, specifically the neurons in the brain. These diseases frequently result in cognitive deterioration, motor dysfunction, and various neurological symptoms. Notable neurodegenerative disorders include Alzheimer's disease, Parkinson's disease, Huntington's disease, and amyotrophic lateral sclerosis (ALS).

Neurodegenerative illnesses commonly exhibit a set of prominent symptoms and characteristics.

1. Neurodegenerative disorders commonly have a gradual and progressive nature, characterized by a sluggish and subtle onset. The symptoms may initially manifest gently and then gradually intensify over a period of time. As the diseases progress, patients may encounter escalating challenges in different

domains of cognitive function, motor control, or both.

2. Neurodegenerative disorders are characterized by the gradual loss of neurons in specific areas of the brain. Neurons play a crucial role in conveying signals within the nervous system, and their deterioration contributes to the symptoms associated with various disorders.

3. Neurodegenerative diseases often involve the aberrant buildup of certain proteins in the brain. As an illustration:

• Alzheimer's Disease is characterized by the buildup of beta-amyloid plaques and tau tangles.

• Parkinson's Disease is characterized by the accumulation of alpha-synuclein in structures known as Lewy bodies.

• Huntington's Disease is characterized by the presence of aggregated mutant huntingtin protein.

4. Inflammation and Oxidative Stress: Inflammatory processes and oxidative stress frequently contribute to the advancement of neurodegenerative disorders. Neuronal death can be facilitated by inflammation, whereas cellular components, including DNA, can be harmed by oxidative stress.

5. Genetic and environmental factors play a role in this. Certain neurodegenerative disorders possess a genetic element, indicating that they can be passed on through inheritance. Nevertheless, the development and progression of many diseases are also influenced by environmental factors, lifestyle choices, and the natural process of aging.

Prevalent Neurodegenerative Disorders:

• Alzheimer's Disease (AD) is defined by the presence of memory loss, cognitive decline, and alterations in behavior. It is the primary cause of dementia.

- Parkinson's Disease (PD) is characterized by the deterioration of dopaminergic neurons, resulting in symptoms associated to movement, such as tremors, rigidity, and bradykinesia (slowed motions).

- Huntington's Disease (HD) is a hereditary condition that leads to gradual deterioration of motor function, cognitive abilities, and mental health.

- Amyotrophic Lateral Sclerosis (ALS) is a neurodegenerative disease that specifically targets motor neurons, resulting in muscle weakening, paralysis, and challenges with speech, swallowing, and breathing.

• Multiple System Atrophy (MSA), Progressive Supranuclear Palsy (PSP), and Corticobasal Degeneration (CBD) are uncommon neurodegenerative conditions that have certain resemblances to Parkinson's disease.

Administration and therapy:

the majority of neurodegenerative diseases do not have a cure. The treatment strategies primarily aim to effectively control symptoms, enhance the overall well-being, and offer assistance to both persons and their caregivers. Continued research is being conducted to gain a deeper understanding of the fundamental causes of these disorders and create specific treatments.

It is crucial to acknowledge that there may have been progress in science and healthcare since my previous update. If you or someone you are acquainted with is impacted by a neurodegenerative disease, it is advisable to seek advice from healthcare experts for the most up-to-date information and tailored direction.

CHAPTE R THREE
Basics of the DASH Diet

The DASH (Dietary Approaches to Stop Hypertension) diet is a specialized eating plan that aims to reduce blood pressure and enhance cardiovascular well-being. The focus is on ingesting nutrient-dense meals that are recognized to have a beneficial effect on blood pressure levels. The following are the fundamental principles of the DASH diet:

1. The DASH diet places great importance on the inclusion of a diverse range of fruits and vegetables, as they are abundant in potassium, magnesium, fiber, and antioxidants. These essential nutrients have the ability to decrease blood pressure and mitigate the likelihood of developing heart disease.

• Strive to consume many portions of fruits and vegetables daily, ensuring a variety of colors and varieties.

2. Whole Grains: Whole grains are a necessary part of the DASH diet, as they supply fiber, vitamins, and minerals. Opt for whole grain alternatives like brown rice, whole wheat bread, oats, quinoa, and barley instead of processed grains.

• Strive to ensure that at least 50% of your grain portions consist of whole grains.

3. Incorporate lean protein sources into your diet, such as fowl, fish, beans, lentils, tofu, and legumes.

• Reduce the amount of red meat you eat and choose lean cuts when you do eat it.

4. Low-Fat Dairy Products: Dairy products are a commendable reservoir of calcium and protein, although they can also contain substantial amounts of saturated fat. The DASH diet advises selecting dairy products that are low in fat or fat-free, including as skim milk, low-fat yogurt, and reduced-fat cheese.

5. If you have lactose intolerance or prefer non-dairy options, fortified soy milk or almond milk can serve as appropriate replacements.

• Include nuts, seeds, and legumes in your diet to increase your intake of protein, beneficial fats, fiber, and minerals.

• Some examples of these foods are almonds, walnuts, chia seeds, flaxseeds, lentils, chickpeas, and black beans.

6. Opt for sources of nutritious fats, such as olive oil, avocado, nuts, and seeds, in moderate amounts.

• Reduce the intake of saturated fats and trans fats commonly found in processed foods, fried foods, and fatty cuts of meat.

7. Decrease Sodium Consumption:
The DASH diet advises decreasing sodium consumption in order to decrease blood pressure. This entails restricting the intake of high-sodium processed foods, canned soups, salty snacks, and sauces.

• Instead, utilize herbs, spices, and other flavorings to season foods without including more sodium.

8. Moderate Alcohol Consumption:

• If you opt to consume alcohol, do it in moderation. For females, this generally refers to consuming a maximum of one alcoholic beverage per day, whereas for males, it refers to consuming a maximum of two alcoholic beverages per day.

• Excessive alcohol use can negatively impact blood pressure and overall health.

The DASH diet is not a rigid regimen, but rather a versatile and well-balanced approach to eating that encourages general health and well-being. It is crucial to acknowledge that the nutritional requirements of each person may differ, and it is recommended to seek guidance from a healthcare expert or registered dietitian, particularly for persons with unique health issues or dietary considerations. In addition, the benefits of the DASH diet for heart health can be further enhanced by including regular physical activity and adopting other good lifestyle practices.

MIND Diet Specifics

The MIND Diet, acronym for "Mediterranean-DASH Diet Intervention for Neurodegenerative Delay," is a specific eating plan aimed at enhancing brain health and maybe lowering the likelihood of neurodegenerative disorders, such as Alzheimer's disease. The diet incorporates components from both the Mediterranean and DASH diets, with an emphasis on foods that are thought to enhance cognitive performance. The MIND Diet consists of precise instructions and components, which are as follows:

1. Focus On Particular Food Items:

• Berries: Specifically, blueberries and strawberries are abundant in antioxidants and have been linked to improvements in cognitive function.

• Leafy greens, such as kale, spinach, and broccoli, should be included in your diet as they are rich in vitamins and minerals.

• Include nuts in your diet, particularly walnuts, as they provide beneficial fats and essential nutrients.

It is recommended to consume fish, particularly fatty fish such as salmon, on a regular basis. This is because fatty fish contains omega-3 fatty acids, which are advantageous for brain health.

• **Whole Grains:** Incorporate whole grains such as quinoa, brown rice, oats, and whole wheat into your diet. These foods are rich in fiber and provide important nutrients.

• Include beans, lentils, and other legumes in your diet to benefit from their protein, fiber, and vitamin content.

• **Poultry:** Consume a moderate amount of poultry, such as chicken or turkey.

• Olive oil should be used as the main source of fat because it is linked to the health of the heart and brain.

• Red wine is recommended in moderation for its possible benefits, while it is optional and not advised for everyone.

2. Foods to Restrict or Eliminate:

• Limit the consumption of red meat, as it is linked to an increased risk of specific health issues.

• Limit the use of butter and margarine, as they contain significant amounts of saturated fats.

• Limit the consumption of cheese, particularly high-fat and processed types.

Limit the consumption of confectionery, pastries, and other high-sugar foods.

3. Meal Planning and Frequency:

- The MIND diet does not provide particular calorie recommendations, but instead focuses on the total nutritional value of food choices.

- It is recommended to consistently include these brain-healthy foods in your meals.

4. Nutritional Goals: The objective of the MIND diet is to supply nutrients that are linked to cognitive health, including antioxidants, omega-3 fatty acids, vitamins, and minerals.

5. The MIND diet promotes adherence and flexibility by accommodating modifications according to individual preferences.

• Research has indicated that even a moderate level of adherence to the MIND diet may be linked to improvements in cognitive function.

6. The scientific foundation of the MIND diet is based on rigorous research, which has established a connection between specific nutrients and dietary patterns and their impact on brain function.

It is crucial to acknowledge that although the MIND diet exhibits potential in enhancing cognitive health, the outcomes may differ among individuals. Furthermore, it is recommended to get guidance from a healthcare expert or a qualified dietitian prior to making substantial modifications to one's dietary habits, particularly for persons with certain health issues or medical problems.

CHAPTER FOUR
Foods to Include

The MIND diet encourages the consumption of specific foods that have been associated with cognitive health and potential benefits for brain function. Here are some key foods to include in the MIND diet:

• **Berries:** Blueberries and strawberries are particularly emphasized due to their high levels of antioxidants, such as anthocyanins, which have been linked to cognitive benefits.

- **Leafy Greens:** Include a variety of leafy green vegetables, such as kale, spinach, collard greens, and broccoli. These are rich in vitamins, minerals, and antioxidants.

- **Nuts:** Walnuts, in particular, are recommended for their omega-3 fatty acids and other nutrients. Other nuts, such as almonds and pistachios, can also be included.

- **Fish:** Fatty fish like salmon, trout, and sardines are excellent sources of omega-3 fatty acids, which have been associated with brain health.

- **Whole Grains:** Choose whole grains over refined grains. Examples include quinoa, brown rice, oats, whole wheat, and barley, providing fiber and essential nutrients.

• **Beans and Legumes:** Incorporate a variety of beans and legumes, such as lentils, chickpeas, black beans, and kidney beans, for their protein, fiber, and nutritional content.

• **Poultry:** Include lean poultry, such as chicken or turkey, as a source of protein. Aim for moderate consumption.

• **Olive Oil:** Use extra virgin olive oil as the primary source of fat in cooking and dressing salads. Olive oil is rich in monounsaturated fats and antioxidants.

- **Wine (Optional):** If desired and appropriate, red wine can be consumed in moderation. The antioxidants, including resveratrol, found in red wine have been associated with potential health benefits.

- **Herbs and Spices:** Use herbs and spices, such as rosemary, thyme, turmeric, and cinnamon, to add flavor to dishes without relying on excess salt.

- **Whole Soy Foods:** Incorporate whole soy foods like tofu and edamame for their protein and potential benefits for brain health.

- **Pomegranate:** Pomegranate is a fruit rich in antioxidants and has been suggested to have potential cognitive benefits.

These foods are chosen based on their nutritional profiles, which include vitamins, minerals, antioxidants, and other compounds that may support cognitive function and protect against neurodegenerative diseases. It's important to note that the MIND diet is not about specific meal plans but rather about incorporating these brain-healthy foods into your overall dietary pattern. Additionally, individual dietary needs and preferences may vary, so it's advisable to consult with a healthcare professional or a registered dietitian for personalized guidance, especially if you have specific health concerns or conditions.

Foods to Avoid

The MIND diet advises restricting the use of specific foods that have been linked to potential detrimental impacts on cognitive well-being. Below are many foods that should be avoided or consumed in limited quantities while following the MIND diet:

- **Red Meat:** Limit the consumption of red meat, including beef and pork. High intake of red meat has been associated with an increased risk of certain health conditions.

- **Butter and Margarine:** Reduce the use of butter and margarine, which are high in saturated fats. Opt for healthier cooking oils like olive oil.

- **Cheese:** Limit the consumption of cheese, especially high-fat and processed varieties. While dairy is included in the diet, it's recommended to choose low-fat options.

- **Sweets and Pastries:** Minimize the intake of sweets, pastries, candies, and other sugary foods. These foods are often high in added sugars, which may have negative effects on overall health.

- **Fried and Processed Foods:** Avoid or limit fried foods and processed snacks, as they can be high in unhealthy fats, sodium, and additives.

- **Fast Food:** Reduce the frequency of fast food consumption, as these meals are often high in saturated fats, sodium, and calories.

- **Whole Fat Dairy:** While moderate consumption of low-fat or fat-free dairy is encouraged, it's advisable to limit the intake of whole-fat dairy products.

- **Pastries and Baked Goods:** Limit the consumption of pastries, cakes, and other baked goods that are often high in refined flour and sugars.

- **High-Sodium Foods:** Reduce the intake of high-sodium foods, including salty snacks, processed meats, and canned soups. Excessive sodium intake can contribute to high blood pressure.

- **Processed and Packaged Foods:** Minimize the consumption of heavily processed and packaged foods, as they may contain preservatives, additives, and unhealthy fats.

- **Trans Fats:** Avoid foods that contain trans fats, which are often found in partially hydrogenated oils. Check ingredient labels for trans fat content.

It's important to note that the MIND diet is not overly restrictive, and occasional indulgences are acceptable. The focus is on incorporating nutrient-dense, brain-healthy foods while being mindful of the intake of less favorable options. Additionally, individual dietary needs may vary, so it's advisable to consult with a healthcare professional or a registered dietitian for personalized guidance, especially if you have specific health concerns or conditions.

CHAPTER FIVE
The MIND Diet and Your Brain

The MIND diet is precisely formulated to enhance brain function and lower the likelihood of neurodegenerative disorders, specifically Alzheimer's disease. The diet is founded on empirical research and includes foods that have been linked to cognitive advantages. The MIND diet can have a beneficial effect on your brain in the following ways:

1. Antioxidant-Rich Foods:

• Berries, especially blueberries and strawberries, are rich in antioxidants that help combat oxidative stress. Oxidative stress is linked to the aging process and neurodegenerative diseases.

2. Omega-3 Fatty Acids:

• Fatty fish, such as salmon, is a source of omega-3 fatty acids. These essential fats play a crucial role in the structure of brain cell membranes and have been associated with cognitive benefits.

3, Leafy Greens and Nutrient Density:

• Leafy green vegetables like kale and spinach are packed with vitamins, minerals, and antioxidants. The nutrient density of these foods supports overall health, including brain function.

4. Whole Grains and Fiber:

• Whole grains provide complex carbohydrates and fiber, contributing to stable blood sugar levels. This helps maintain energy levels and supports overall cognitive function.

5. Nuts and Healthy Fats:

• Nuts, especially walnuts, are rich in healthy fats, including omega-3 fatty acids. Healthy fats are essential for brain health and function.

6. Lean Proteins: Lean proteins from sources like poultry, beans, and legumes provide amino acids necessary for the production of neurotransmitters, supporting communication between brain cells.

7. Olive Oil and Monounsaturated Fats: Extra virgin olive oil, a staple in the MIND diet, is a source of monounsaturated fats. These fats are associated with cardiovascular health, which is closely linked to brain health.

8. Reduced Inflammatory Foods:

• The MIND diet recommends limiting the intake of red meat and processed foods, which may contribute to inflammation. Chronic inflammation is associated with various health conditions, including neurodegenerative diseases.

9. Moderate Alcohol Consumption:

• Red wine, consumed in moderation, is suggested for its potential cardiovascular benefits and antioxidant content. However, it's important to note that excessive alcohol consumption can have negative effects on health.

10. Mindful Food Choices:

• The MIND diet encourages mindful food choices, promoting a balanced and varied diet that includes a wide range of nutrients beneficial for brain health.

Studies on the MIND diet have demonstrated encouraging links to cognitive function and a decreased susceptibility to Alzheimer's disease. Following the MIND diet has been associated with a deceleration in cognitive decline and a reduced occurrence of neurodegenerative disorders.

It is crucial to acknowledge that nutrition is merely one component in preserving brain function. Additional lifestyle factors, such as consistent physical exercise, cognitive engagement, sufficient rest, and general state of health, also have a role in cognitive performance. Prior to implementing substantial modifications to your dietary regimen, particularly if you own specific health conditions, it is prudent to get advice from healthcare professionals or certified dietitians for tailored recommendations.

Planning and Implementing the MIND Diet

Developing and executing the MIND diet entails integrating nutrients that promote brain health into your regular dietary routine. Below are a series of stages to guide you in the process of planning and implementing the MIND diet:

- Acquaint yourself with the MIND Diet Guidelines: o Comprehend the fundamental principles of the MIND diet, which prioritize the consumption of berries, leafy greens, nuts, fish, whole grains, and olive oil. Acquaint yourself with the kind of meals that you should restrict or refrain from consuming.

- Evaluate your present dietary patterns to determine areas where you can conform to the principles of the MIND diet. Make a record of the meals you now eat that align with the MIND recommendations and identify any that may require modification.

- Develop a weekly meal plan by strategically selecting meals that include foods that align with the MIND diet. Incorporate a diverse selection of fruits, vegetables, complete grains, lean proteins, and nutritious fats. It is advisable to utilize herbs and spices to enhance the taste of food rather than relying on excessive amounts of salt.

• Incorporate berries into your snacks and dinners. These fruits can be consumed in their natural state, incorporated into yogurt, blended into smoothies, or utilized as toppings for cereals and sweets.

• Select whole grains: o Choose whole grains such brown rice, quinoa, oats, and whole wheat bread. Replace processed grains with whole grains in your meals.

• Integrate fatty fish into your diet: o Consume fatty fish such as salmon, trout, or sardines at least twice a week. These fish contain high levels of omega-3 fatty acids.

• Consume nuts as a snack, especially walnuts, for a nourishing and fulfilling choice.

• Utilize olive oil for culinary purposes: o Opt for extra virgin olive oil while cooking or as a dressing for salads. It is a fundamental component of the MIND diet and a provider of nutritious monounsaturated fats.

• Restrict the intake of red meat and processed meals by decreasing their frequency of consumption. Choose low-fat protein sources such as poultry, beans, and lentils.

• Incorporate a diverse selection of beans and legumes into your meals. They include high levels of protein, fiber, and other minerals.

• Maintain proper hydration: o Consume ample amounts of water throughout the day to ensure proper hydration. Restrict the intake of sugary beverages and choose water, herbal teas, or infused water instead.

• Implement Portion Control: o Exercise awareness of portion proportions to uphold a well-balanced and nutritious diet. Excessive consumption, even of nourishing foods, can have a negative effect on general well-being.

• Embrace Adaptability and Appreciate Diversity: o The MIND diet offers flexibility, accommodating a wide range of foods and flavors. Discover novel culinary creations and savor the wide range of nourishing dishes.

• Seek advice from an expert: If you have certain health issues or unique dietary requirements, it is advisable to speak with a healthcare professional or a qualified dietitian. They are capable of offering tailored advice that takes into account your specific situation.

It is important to keep in mind that the process of adopting a new eating pattern requires patience and making progressive changes over time. It is crucial to implement modifications that are both enduring and pleasurable for you. In addition, integrating other healthy lifestyle habits, such as consistent physical exercise and cognitive engagement, enhances the advantages of the MIND diet in promoting total brain well-being.

CHAPTER SIX
MIND Diet and Age-Related Cognitive Decline

The MIND diet has been studied for its potential impact on age-related cognitive decline and the risk of developing neurodegenerative diseases, particularly Alzheimer's disease. While research in this area is ongoing, several studies have suggested a positive association between adherence to the MIND diet and cognitive health. Here are key findings related to the MIND diet and age-related cognitive decline:

• **Reduced Cognitive Decline:**

Research has shown that individuals who closely adhere to the MIND diet may experience a slower rate of cognitive decline as they age compared to those who do not follow the diet as closely. This includes a decline in cognitive functions such as memory, attention, and executive function.

- **Lower Risk of Alzheimer's Disease:**

Several studies have reported a potential association between adherence to the MIND diet and a reduced risk of developing Alzheimer's disease. One study found that individuals with high adherence to the MIND diet had a significantly lower risk of Alzheimer's disease compared to those with lower adherence.

• Protective Role of Specific Foods:

Certain components of the MIND diet, such as berries and leafy greens, have been individually associated with cognitive benefits. For example, the high antioxidant content of berries and the nutrient density of leafy greens are believed to contribute to neuroprotection.

• Omega-3 Fatty Acids and Brain Health:

The MIND diet includes fatty fish as a source of omega-3 fatty acids, which have been linked to improved cognitive function and a potential protective role against cognitive decline.

• Impact on Inflammation and Oxidative Stress:

The MIND diet's emphasis on antioxidant-rich foods may help mitigate inflammation and oxidative stress, which are processes associated with aging and neurodegenerative diseases.

• Observational Studies:

Observational studies tracking the dietary habits of individuals over time have provided evidence supporting the MIND diet's potential to positively influence cognitive health in aging populations.

It's important to note that while these findings are promising, the MIND diet is not a guaranteed preventive measure, and individual responses may vary. Additionally, factors such as genetics, overall lifestyle, and other health conditions can influence cognitive health.

Adopting the MIND diet, along with other healthy lifestyle practices such as regular physical activity, adequate sleep, and mental stimulation, may contribute to overall well-being and reduce the risk of age-related cognitive decline. Before making significant changes to your diet, especially if you have specific health concerns, it's advisable to consult with healthcare professionals or registered dietitians for personalized guidance based on your individual circumstances.

Overcoming Obstacles to MIND Diet Adherence

Adhering to any diet plan can be challenging, and the MIND diet is no exception. However, there are strategies to overcome common obstacles and make it easier to incorporate brain-healthy eating habits into your lifestyle. Here are some tips to help you overcome obstacles to MIND diet adherence:

- **Gradual Changes:** Instead of making drastic changes all at once, consider making gradual adjustments to your eating habits. Start by incorporating a few MIND diet principles into your meals and snacks, and then expand from there.

- **Meal Planning:** Plan your meals and snacks in advance. This can help you ensure that you have the necessary ingredients on hand and reduce the temptation to opt for less healthy food choices.

- **Batch Cooking:** Cook larger quantities of MIND diet-friendly meals and freeze portions for later. This can save time and make it easier to stick to your dietary goals, especially on busy days.

- **Include Favorites:** Identify MIND diet-friendly foods that you already enjoy and incorporate them into your meals. This can make the dietary transition more enjoyable and sustainable.

- **Explore New Recipes:** Experiment with new recipes that align with the MIND diet. There are many creative and delicious ways to prepare brain-healthy foods. Trying new dishes can keep your meals interesting and prevent boredom.

- **Smart Substitutions:** Make smart substitutions in your existing recipes. For example, replace saturated fats with healthier fats like olive oil, and choose whole grains over refined grains.

- **Mindful Eating:** Practice mindful eating by paying attention to your body's hunger and fullness cues. This can help you avoid overeating and make more conscious food choices.

- **Social Support:** Share your dietary goals with friends, family, or a support group. Having a supportive network can provide encouragement and motivation to stay on track.

- **Nutrient-Dense Snacks:** Keep nutrient-dense snacks readily available. Having healthy options like nuts, fresh fruits, or cut vegetables on hand can prevent reaching for less nutritious snacks when hungry.

- **Stay Hydrated:**

Drink plenty of water throughout the day. Staying hydrated is essential for overall health and can help curb unnecessary snacking.

- **Flexibility:**

Be flexible and forgiving with yourself. Understand that occasional deviations from the MIND diet are normal. Aim for consistency rather than perfection.

- **Education and Awareness:**

Educate yourself about the nutritional benefits of MIND diet foods. Understanding how specific foods contribute to brain health can reinforce your commitment to the diet.

• **Celebrate Small Wins:**

Acknowledge and celebrate your achievements, no matter how small. Recognizing your progress can boost your confidence and motivation.

• **Professional Guidance:**

If needed, seek guidance from a registered dietitian or healthcare professional. They can provide personalized advice based on your health status and dietary preferences.

Remember that dietary changes are a journey, and it's okay to progress at your own pace. By making gradual adjustments and finding ways to make the MIND diet enjoyable, you can overcome obstacles and create sustainable habits that support brain health.

Physical Activity and the MIND Diet

Engaging in physical activity is essential for promoting overall health, including the health of the brain. Regular exercise, when combined with a brain-healthy diet such as the MIND diet, can improve cognitive performance, lower the risk of neurodegenerative disorders, and promote general well-being. The synergy between physical exercise and the MIND diet is as follows:

- **Cardiovascular Health:** Both physical activity and adherence to the MIND diet have been linked to enhanced cardiovascular health. The health of the cardiovascular system is intricately connected to the health of the brain, as an optimal blood circulation facilitates the transportation of oxygen and essential nutrients to the brain.

- **Blood Flow to the Brain:** Regular physical activity enhances the circulation of blood, a crucial factor in sustaining good brain performance. Sufficient blood circulation supplies oxygen and nutrients to the cells of the brain and aids in the elimination of waste substances.

- Physical activity has demonstrated neuroprotective properties, safeguarding the integrity and functionality of the brain. When combined with the MIND diet's emphasis on foods that are high in antioxidants, this can help safeguard the brain from oxidative stress.

• **Cognitive Benefits:** Both exercise and the MIND diet have separately shown cognitive advantages. When combined, these substances can have a synergistic impact, enhancing cognitive function and potentially lowering the likelihood of cognitive decline.

• **Weight control:** Engaging in regular physical exercise aids with weight control, and sustaining a healthy weight is linked to a reduced likelihood of developing chronic illnesses, including those that impact the brain. The MIND diet, which prioritizes meals that are rich in nutrients, supports a strategy for maintaining a healthy weight.

• **Enhanced Emotional State and Alleviation of Stress:** Physical activity is recognized for its ability to enhance emotional well-being and alleviate stress, both of which can have a good effect on cognitive health. The MIND diet incorporates foods that have mood-enhancing and stress-reducing qualities, such as omega-3 fatty acids, which can contribute to improved mental well-being.

7. **Increased Neuroplasticity:** Engaging in physical activity has been associated with enhanced neuroplasticity, which refers to the

brain's capacity to adapt and establish new connections. Integrating physical activity with a diet that is high in nutrients can enhance the conditions necessary for neuroplasticity and cognitive flexibility.

• **Joint Support:** Regular exercise promotes the preservation of joint health and flexibility. This can promote a dynamic lifestyle, enabling individuals to participate in diverse forms of physical activity that enhance overall well-being.

• A balanced lifestyle can be achieved by incorporating both the MIND diet and regular physical activity, which together contribute to a comprehensive and well-rounded approach to overall well-being. This strategy encompasses various dimensions of health, encompassing diet, physical fitness, and mental well-being.

• **Personalized Approach:** Take into account your own tastes and physical capabilities while integrating physical activity into your daily regimen. Engaging in activities such as walking, running, swimming, cycling, and strength training can all enhance the overall advantages of leading an active lifestyle.

It is crucial to acknowledge that the precise guidelines for physical activity can differ depending on an individual's health condition, age, and level of fitness. Prior to commencing a new workout plan or implementing substantial modifications to your diet, it is prudent to get tailored advise from healthcare specialists or fitness experts.

By integrating the MIND diet with consistent physical exercise, you establish a harmonious strategy to enhance your entire health and well-being, encompassing cognitive performance and brain health.

Conclusion

To summarize, the MIND diet presents a hopeful strategy for enhancing brain health and potentially decreasing the likelihood of age-related cognitive decline and neurodegenerative disorders. The MIND diet is based on the ideas of the Mediterranean and DASH diets, and focuses on consuming nutrient-rich foods that have been linked to improved cognitive function.

• The MIND diet emphasizes the consumption of berries, leafy greens, nuts, fish, whole grains, and olive oil, while restricting the consumption of red meat, butter, and processed foods. The diet is specifically formulated to supply vital nutrients, including antioxidants, omega-3 fatty acids, and vitamins, that are needed for supporting cognitive function.

• Studies indicate that following the MIND diet is linked to a deceleration in cognitive decline, a lower likelihood of developing Alzheimer's disease, and possible neuroprotective benefits. Furthermore, integrating the MIND diet with consistent physical activity, a well-rounded lifestyle, and other healthful practices amplifies its influence on overall wellness.

• Overcoming barriers to adhering to the MIND diet requires implementing progressive modifications, engaging in meal planning, integrating preferred foods, experimenting with novel recipes, and requesting assistance from social networks. Flexibility, awareness, and acknowledging little victories are crucial elements in effectively establishing and maintaining brain-healthy dietary habits.

It is crucial to acknowledge that there might be variations in how individuals respond to the MIND diet. Factors such as genetics, overall lifestyle, and other health issues contribute to cognitive health. Prior to implementing substantial modifications to your dietary or physical fitness regimen, it is recommended to get advice from healthcare specialists or certified dietitians for tailored counsel.

By integrating the concepts of the MIND diet with a dynamic and harmonious lifestyle, individuals can proactively preserve cognitive function, enhance brain health, and cultivate general well-being as they age.

THE END